CANDIDA ALBICANS

Step by Step to Defeat Candida Overgrowth

CHEN BEN ASHER

CANDIDA ALBICANS

Step by Step to Defeat Candida Overgrowth

www.mor-nutrition4life.com

TABLE OF CONTENT

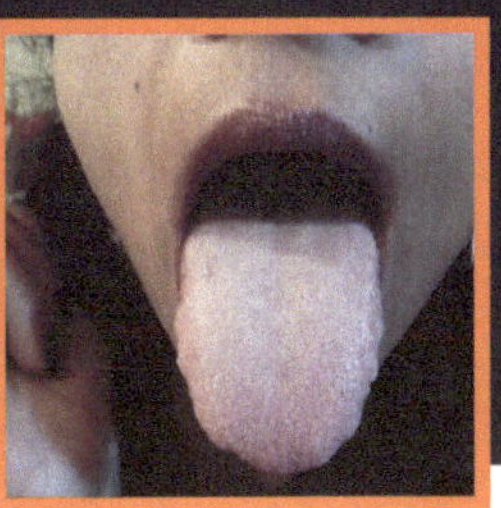

True, we all have trillions of bacteria, fungi and parasites, both outside and inside our bodies. These living organisms are inhibiting in our digestive tract, making up the normal "microflora." These living organisms play a supportive role in the health of the colon by helping to synthesize vitamins, degrade toxins, and produce natural antibiotics .

They are opportunistic living creatures, who colonize in many parts of the body, particularly the gut and genitourinary tracts, with one goal in "mind": to survive and thrive. Their ability to meet this goal is depends on our overall health. If we are healthy and balanced nutritionally, chances are they will not thrive.

In cases when we find yeast infection, the delicate bacterial balance is interfering. It can create great damage, weakening our immune system leading to a disease by effecting multiple body systems. This "domino" reaction reduces cellular metabolism. Our kidnies and liver detoxification will be compromised, joint discomfort aches and pain will occur, and brain function will decrease. As well as reduction in food absorption due to waste production by these organism, causing inflammation in the intestinal wall.

In a worse case scenario where the colonies are thriving and prolifering a biofilm will be created (a closely packed microbial communities of cells), more damage on the cellular level accure which makes it even harder and longer to treat and reduce the chronic infection.

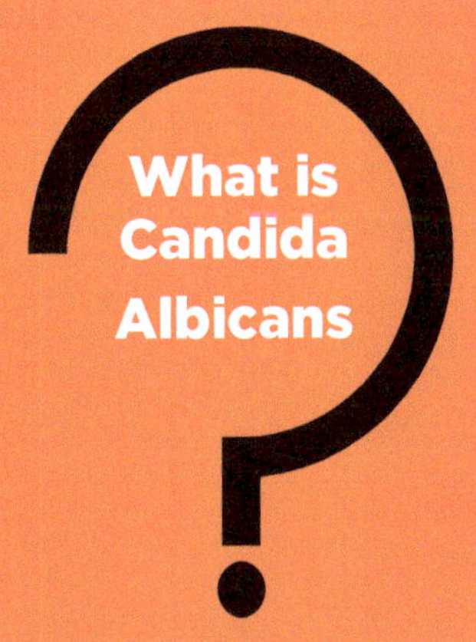

What is Candida Albicans

There are over 20 species of candida that can cause infections in human. The most common one is Candida Albicans.

Candida albicans is the most prevalent fungal species of the human microbioti. It is a yeast-like fungus, that is found in small amounts in the mouth and intestines within each one of us. The main function of candida is to help with digestion and nutrient absorption.

When conditions permit it, and if these yeast organisms are allowed to grow with no control, the internal bacteria ratio will change and the balance will be shift, resulting in intestinal candidiasis or what has been called "yeast overgrowth". Yeast overgrowth, may lead to break down of the wall of the intestines and penetrate the bloodstream and from there throughout the body. During this process the yeast change to a fungus form, which creates a faster process of proliferation and colonies are formed. This process releases bio-waste and toxins which lead to gut permeability, "leaky gut" and IBS (Irritable bowel syndrome). Gut candida infection may interfere with the absorption of CoQ10 as well as an increase in the likelihood of the development of food sensitivities and GI distress and disorders

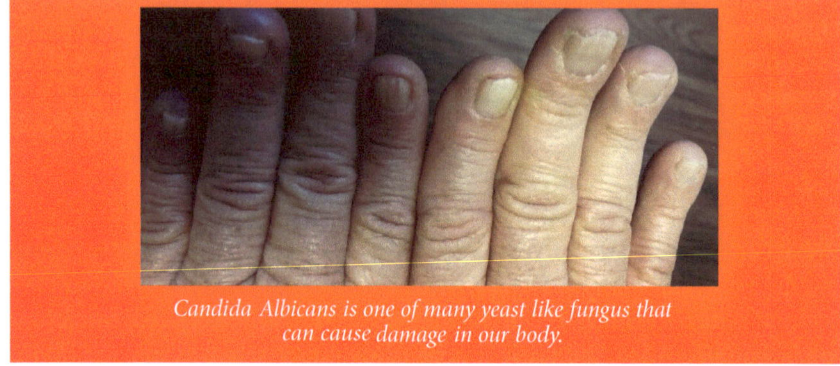

Candida Albicans is one of many yeast like fungus that can cause damage in our body.

Candida albicans overgrowth, along with stress, compromises the nutrition and will decreased the immune system response to the point of developing a disease. At this point, the candida fungus is developing biofilm which protect the candida from the immune system attack by its cellular membrane. In simple words, the immune system is losing the battle against candida which can exhaust you, and leave you prone to potential diseases.

Candida fungi are anaerobic. Meaning, they do not need oxygen to metabolize and survive. This issue, the likelihood, of potential growth of cancer cells, which thrive in low oxygen environment.

DO NOT IGNORE IT!

There are also numerous other health problems possible that are related to candida overgrowth that affect not just the digestive system but can also affect the brain, nervous system, joints, and skin. Also the liver can become overloaded with stored toxins, which greatly impairs its ability to work as a detoxifier, and this can lead to chronic disease

COMMON SYMPTOMS THAT MAY BE ASSOCIATED WITH YEAST OVERGROWTH AND/OR CANDIDA INFECTION

On the digestive system:	On the brain:
 • Gas • Bloating • Cramping • Diarrhea or constipation • Heartburn • Reflux	• Confused thinking • "Brain fog" • Impaired memory • Depression • Moodiness • Irritability • Trouble concentrating • Anxiety/panic attack
On the skin:	**Other systems:**
• Rashes • Itches • Hives • Itchy patches on the skin • "jock itch"	• Malaise • Sweet cravings • Alcohol need • Sore gums • Fatigue • Allergies (food and/or environmental) • Vaginal itch or discharge • Frequent bladder infections • Thrush in the mouth • Severity of the infection • Chemical Sensitivities
On the Hormonal system:	
• Menstrual irregularities • Decreased libido • PMS • Breast Swelling • Decreased sex drive	

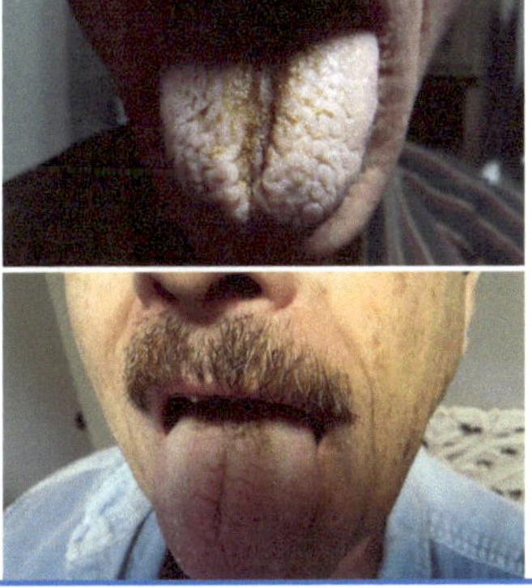

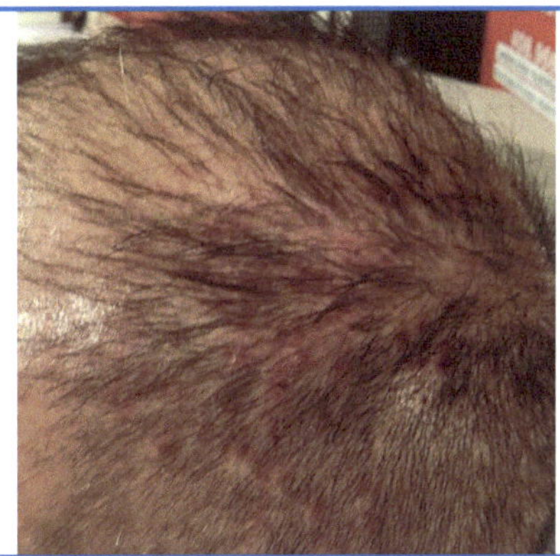

SYMPTOMS & PROGRESSION

Thrush	Sugar and Alcohol craving	Alcoholism
Sore Throat	Migraines	Asthma
Bloating and Gas	Anxiety, Depression	Addison's Disease
Constipation and Diarrhea in rotation	Fatigue	Chronic Fatigue Syndrome
Ear ache	Vaginitis	Leaky Gut, IBS
Rashes and/or Itches	Foggy Thinking	Depression and Anxiety Disorders
Bad Breath	Skin Infection	Psoriasis
Blurred Vision	Hyperactivity, Irritability	Arthritis
	Recurrent bladder infections	
	Sinus Inflammation	Cancer
	Dizziness	
	Insomnia	
	Low Sex Drive	
	Ear ache	
	Chronic Pain	
	Muscle Weakness	

Progression Of Candida

Infection → Reach the Blood → Tissue Damage → Disease

Most individuals will face multiple symptoms in different systems which make it even harder to locate the root cause of a potential candida. If you have several of the signs and symptoms of a Candida infection then it is very likely that the Candida fungus has escaped your gut and is now loose in your body, causing long-term damage to your health.

CONTRIBUTION FACTORS FOR CANDIDA

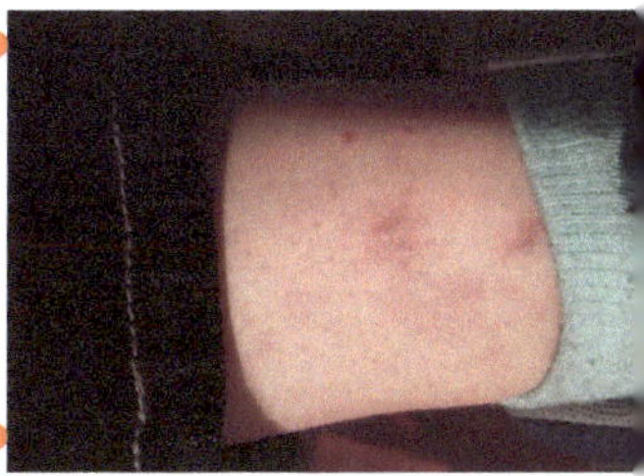

At least some of these factors can be found in most people's daily lives, thus leading to wonder what are symptoms of candida?

- Repeated use of antibiotics and/or steroids
- Immune Suppressive medications for organ transplant
- Chemotherapy
- Intravenous, urinary or other catheters
- Infections that appear on skin and nails like athlete's foot or toenail fungus
- Infections of urinary tract, vagina as well as itching in those places
- Chronic stress and fatigue
- Diet high in simple sugars
- Diet consisting of refined carbs
- Overweight
- Alcohol
- Oral contraceptive use
- Diabetes
- Weak immune system

- Pregnancy
- Catching it from a sex partner who has yeast infection
- Autoimmune diseases like "Hashimoto's thyroiditis, rheumatoid arthritis, 1
- 1 ulcerative colitis, lupus, psoriasis, scleroderma, or multiple sclerosis"
- Poor memory, various difficulties in concentrating, ADHD (Attention deficit
- Hyperactivity disorder), ADD (Atten tion-Deficit Disorder), brain fog
- Problems with skin like eczema, hives, psoriasis, rashes
- Mood swings, depression, irritability, anxiety
- Sessional allergies or itchy ears

AVAILABLE TESTS

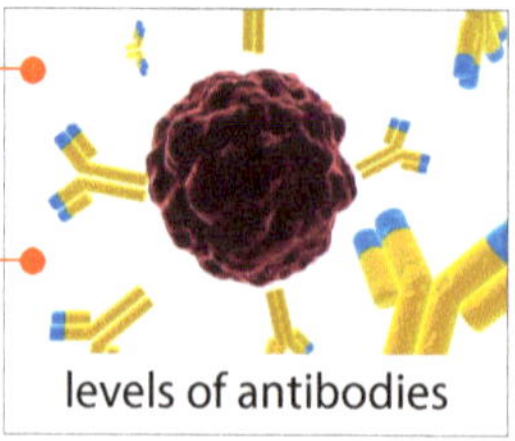

levels of antibodies

If you suspect candida yeast overgrowth you will want to test for it so you could take proper steps to lower the potential damage of candida infection on your health.

> A simple blood test will check the levels of antibodies (IgG, IgA, IgM) to the candida.

- Levels of IgG reflect past and present infection
- Levels of IgM reflect present infection
- Levels of IgA reflect present infection of the mucosal lining of the body

Candida overgrowth can be easily determined in special laboratories without problems.

For a more concrete diagnosis also **comprehensive stool test**, **urine-organic test** and **gut dysbiosis test (one or all)** might be performed. **Stool testing** allows to detect candida in the colon or lower intestines, as well as other organism like parasites, fungi and bacteria. Reducing the levels of candida infection does not necessary reduce levels of harmful bacteria like: **Proteus mirabilis, Klebsiella pneumoniae, Enterobacter cloacae, Campylobacter species, Citrobacter species, Clostridium difficile, Staphylococcus aureus, Various streptococcus species,** that can infect the small intestines. The bad bacteria treatment plan is slightly different from yeast infection.

Organic acids check also the bio-waste products and toxins due to candida infection.

Results of any of the suggested tests will determine the yeast species as well as treatment

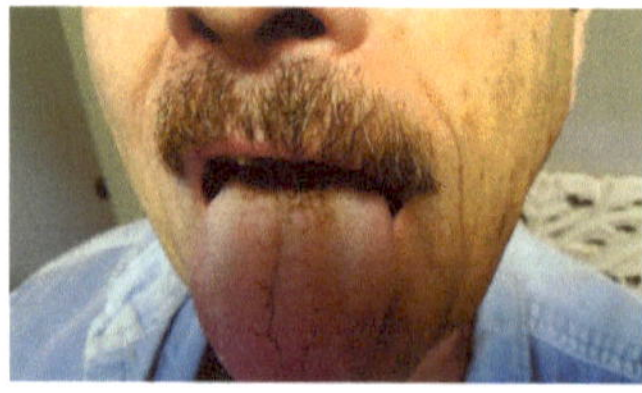

Candida complicated due to chromogenic bacteria and/or staining from exogenous sources. Individuals may experience gagging sensation, altered taste or halitosis

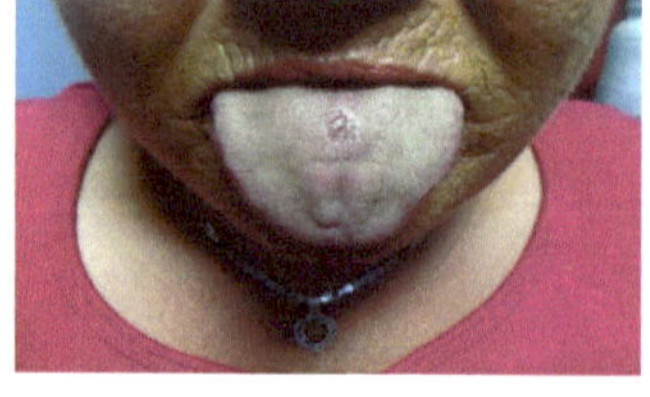

Candidiasis Thrush - an infection in the mouth creating a whitish film on the palate, tongue, and inside cheeks. When thrush extends into the throat it causes Esophagitis.

CANDIDA - CANCER CONNECTION

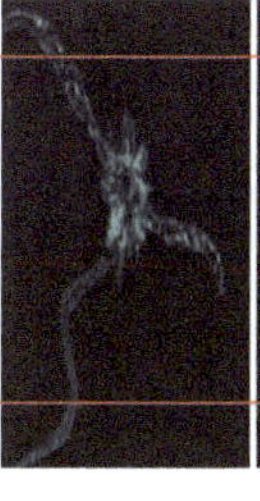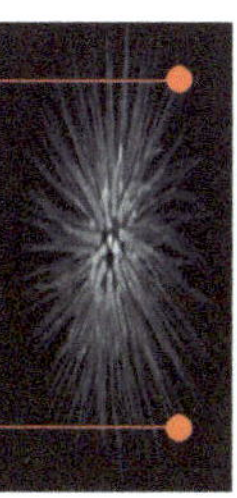

There is an increasing concern about the relation between microbial nfection such as candida albicans and cancer. Candida albican infection increases the risk of carcinogenesis and metastasis. In fact, most recent studies show that candida albican infections are capable of promoting cancer by several bio-mechanisms, among them is Triggering inflammation, inducing of TH17 response (T helper cells which function as a mediators of the cellular immune response against extracellular bacteria, fungus and autoimmunity) and molecular mimicry.

Food can change your cells environment when parasitical fungus challenging the immune system and increasing its activity and therefore, compromising and weakening, particularly chronic infections which may initiate cell division abnormalities that lead to cancer cells in some individuals by two different mechanisms:

1 Secretion of degradative enzymes by the candida fungi that affect aspartic proteases (enzymes that breaks proteins into small pieces), which may digest the epithelial cell surface components. This allows the physical movement of the hyphae into, or between the host cells. In simple words: the fungus cytoplasm (a thick solution that fills each cell with water, salt and proteins, and is enclosed by the cell membrane) is surrounded by a rigid wall which separates it from the external environment which allows the candida fungi to proliferate.

2 Induction of the epithelial cell endocytosis which stimuli keratinocyte cells (cells that form a protective barrier between the nerves and the skin layer that prevents the entry of foreigners and infections into the cells). Candida albican has been shown to act as a promoter for carcinogenesis cells.

Candida Yeast → Candida → Fungus → Infection → In-lammation → Cancer

---

DON'T IGNORE CANDIDA

No doubt, bacteria and viruses stimulate cancerdevelopment or progression. Candida albican is no different. Taking control over Candida yeast infections may prevent the pro-tumor effect of the fungal species.

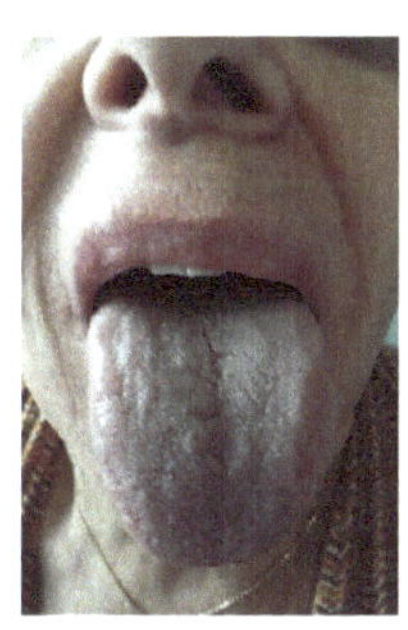

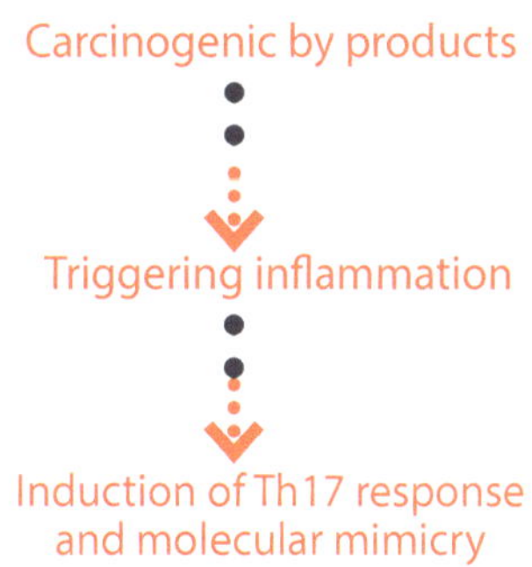

CANDIDA - FOOD SENSITIVITY ALLERGY CONNECTION

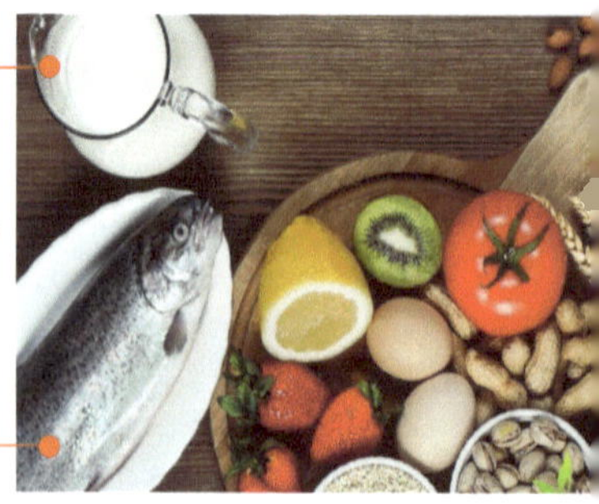

Because Candida albicans is a naturally occurring organism in the intestinal tract of the human body, Candidiasis occurs everywhere.

Over 70 % of a body's immunity is in the digestive tract. Any imbalances will affect your body immediately, reducing the possibility to fight even the smallest infections. Food sensitivity and food allergies that have not been detected, eliminated and supportedby nutritional changes and supplements, will create inflammatory and immunopathology reactions. This will affect the intestinal integrity, damaging the intestinal lining tissues caused by the mycelia of the candida fungus and candida metabolism.

Candida toxins and inflammation that have been produced in the gut such as zymosan and arabinitol are associated with the psoriasis, brain, nervous system, immune system, memory retention, hormone disturbance, fatigue, depression, rheumatoid arthritis, thyroiditis and even celiac desease. Not to say, gut symbiosis, Irritable Bowel Syndrome (IBS), leaky gut, colitis, chron's desease, nutritional deficiencies and more.

Elimination diet alone will not reduce these inflammatory reactions, tissue damage and recovery.

A nutritional holistic approach needs to be included in your journey to take control of candida albicans.

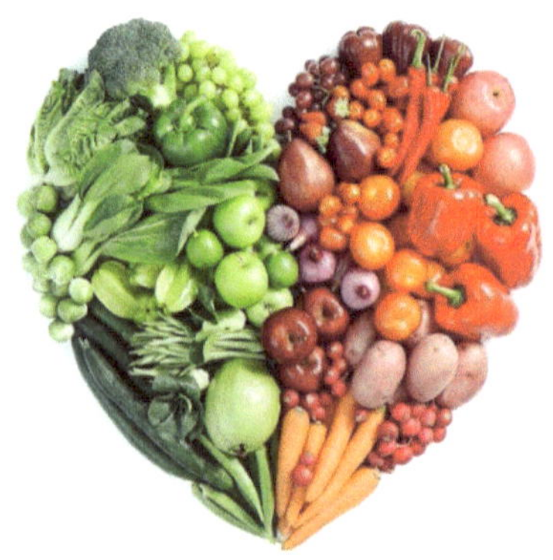

THE CANDIDA NUTRITIONAL PROTOCOL

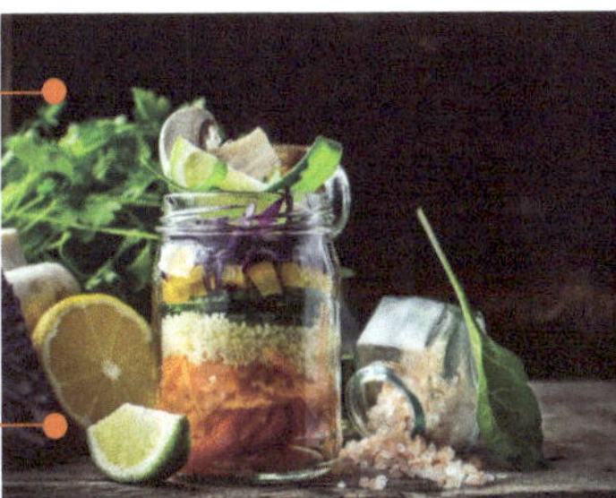

Nutritional Support to Control Candida Overgrowth

If you have candida yeast overgrowth, you must take the right steps to control the yeast-fungus damage and bring it back to a controlled and healthy equilibrium volume. This program requires your personal efforts, nutritional and dietary hanges, supplementation and in some cases even medication.

You are the SUCCESS of this PROGRAM.

It's important not to attempt to self-treat this conditions.

It is a challenging, and it requires a learning curve, care and support from an experienced health professional.

Dietary changes are NEVER easy!

However, diet is an essential and integral part of the process. It's ONLY one part of the puzzle of reducing the yeast-fungus volume.

The healing process: supporting your immune system, supporting the gut tract, balancing energy production, closing nutritional gaps of micro and macro nutrients are all part of the following holistic approach to reducing severity of your yeast-fungus levels.

THREE STEPS – THREE PHASES

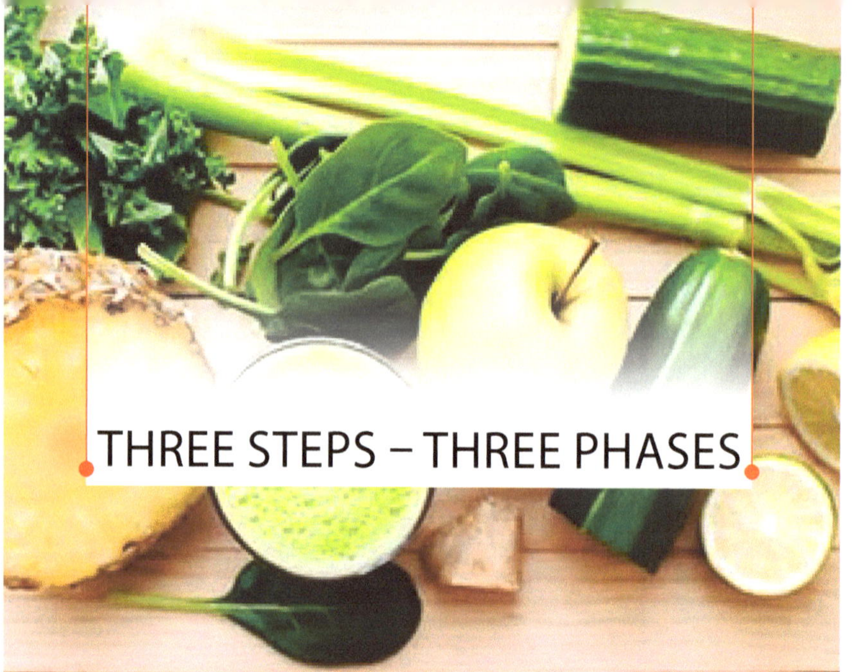

YEAST-FUNGUS REDUCTION VOLUME

Elimination ☐   60 or 90 days ☐   Starting Date

In the next days, you will eliminate any foods that feed the yeast-fungus overgrowth. These are live organisms that depended like us, on food to survive.

Candida thrive on sugar foods by using the carbon source for growth and proliferation from all foods that break down to be sugars. Food like: fruits, grains, starchy vegetables, beans, legumes, mushrooms, alcohol and fermented foods will support the proliferation process of yeast. An excess of sugar foods (even if it's considered to be healthy), will lower the immune system capability of fighting, any disease including fighting candida. The goal is to be on a very low carbohydrates diet, supporting the immune system to produce neutrophils (type of WBC) against candida.

Don't choose to be on a Sugar Free diet. It will lower your blood sugar, create ketosis which will suppress the immune system.

Small amounts of carbohydrates from diverse food will support the first phase of reducing candida volume.

General Guides:

a You want to eat at least 3 meals a day: breakfast, lunch and dinner and 2 small meals (snacks)

b Eat to be satisfied (no worries about your weight scale)

c Drink plenty of water, herbal teas

" SugarpromotesCandida RapidgrowthandSpread **"**

WHAT TO AVOID EATING IN THE FIRST PHASE

1 **Fresh fruits** up to 1/4 cup as serving size twice a day (better to AVOID completely in the first 60 days)

No Melons: Watermelon, honeydew and, especially, cantaloupe (high in mold and sugar)

2 **Carbohydrate foods**

a. Healthy carbohydrates reduced to no more than ½ cup as a serving size

b. Please choose low glycemic index carbohydrate foods. Which are more slowly digested, absorbed and metabolized and cause a lower and slower rise in blood glucose and insulin levels.

3 No refined Sugar Foods (even not a bit!)

4 No Grains - All refined or whole grains, breads, baked goods, products made with flour which turn to sugar. Avoid grains like: wheat, rice, quinoa, soy, corn, barley, kamut, Millet, Teff

5 **No processed foods** (hidden sources of sugar)

I. Too many hidden sugar substance like: Dextrose, Fruit Juice Concentrate, Glucose, Malt syrup, Maltose, Molasses, Sucrose, lactose, Beet sugar, High-fructose corn syrup (HFCS), Evaporated cane juice, rice sugar, glycogen, glucose, mannitol, sorbitol, galactose, mono-saccharides and polysaccharides. Also avoid honey, molasses, maple sugar, date sugar and turbinado sugar.

II. No "monosodium glutamate"

III. No Vegetables Oils – This are polyunsaturated fat. Oxidize quickly. Contain hydrogenerated fats or trans fatty acids which do not support the immune system to fight yeast. Instead you want to use saturated fat like virgin coconut oil (VCO) or even grass-fed lard, support the immune system, your intestines, it is Anti-bacterial, anti-viral and anti-fungal

IV. NO Food Additive or food coloring

V. NO Canned or Boxed foods of any kind

6

VI. No Ketchup - most ketchup contains about 4 grams of sugar per 1 teaspoon. Make your own tomatoes sauce or buy sugar free solution. There is nothing like slices of juicy fresh tomatoes on an hamburger

VII. No Dried Fruits - Raisins, apricots, dates, prunes, figs and pineapple. Dried fruit is not as nutritious as fresh fruit. Dried fruit contains hidden sugar per serv ing. A quarter cup of raisins contains 7 teaspoons of sugar. Better to eat 1 serving of fresh fruit to regulate your blood sugar and control candida. However, in this first phase, you want to reduce even fresh fruits to ¼ cup as serving size

VIII. No Soft Drinks, Fruit Juices – are high in their sugar levels. Mainly, high fructose corn syrup (HFCS), fructose and aspartame (if it's "diet"), sweet soda drinks also con tain carbonic and phosphoric acids as well as halogens like fluorides in their mix -- all of which only works to greatly acidify your body which supports candida spread. HFCS also contains mercury and also contains poisonous chemicals like glutaraldehyde which is normally used as a poisonous industrial cleaner.

IX. No Sweeteners – no aspartame, sucralose or saccharine. These additives are excitotoxins that damage our central nerve system, produce methanol which stress internal organs like our liver and kidneys, suppress the thymus which lower your body ability to detoxify and support the fight against candida.

X. NO Processed or smoked meats like: sausages, hot dogs, corned beef, pastrami, smoked fish, ham, cheeses and bacon. These often contain sugars, starches, and additives.

XI. No Malt (requires reading labels)

XII. Malt products: Malted milk drinks, cereals and candy. (Malt is a sprouted grain that is kiln-dried and used in the preparation of man processed foods and beverages.)

XIII. No Vinegar and food with vinegar made like: mayonnaise, pickles, pickled foods, mustard and relish.

> Please Note: Some people will do fine with raw apple cider vinegar which is unpasteurized and unfiltered (use Bragg's and Eden's)

7 NO Edible Mushrooms – mushrooms are a type of fungi, morels and truffles

8 Fats and oils – AVOID Margarine, shortening, processed oils, prepared salad dressings, spreads and sauces, mayonnaise

9 No Leftovers: Molds grow in leftover food unless it's properly refrigerated. Use better freezing methods

10 NO Alcohol – Wines and beers. Most alcoholic beverage are contaminated with yeast and high in their sugar content which will feed your candida.

HOW DO YOU CALCULATE HOW MANY TEASPOONS OF SUGAR ARE IN THE PRODUCT YOU WANT TO EAT?

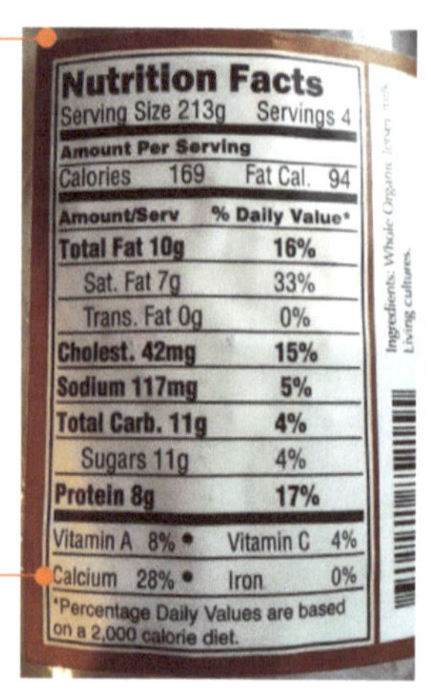

Look at your food labels. In this example the product label has 11 grams of sugar, you have to multiply the number of grams (11g) by the number of serving (4) to get the total grams of sugar in the product:

11 x 4 = 44grams of sugar.

4 grams of sugar equals one teaspoon.

So, we have in this example 11 (44/4=11) teaspoons of sugar

Would you eat 11 teaspoons of sugar?

WHAT CAN YOU EAT?

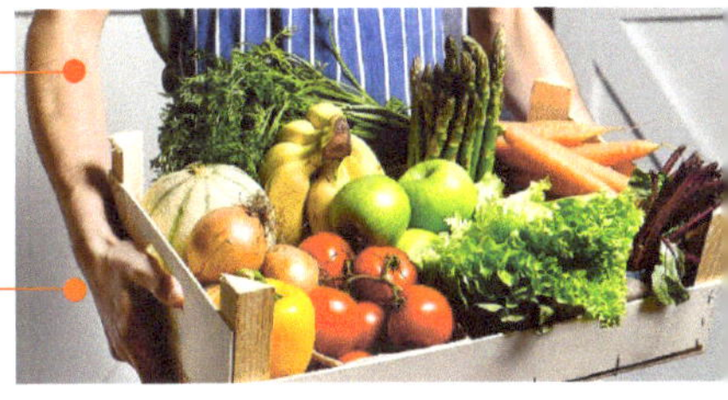

1 **Vegetables** – no limitation (Organic, fresh, non GMO and local if possible) Cooked, boiled and grilled vegetables. Cooked vegetables will support your gut tract to heal faster.

- Try to limit all raw vegetables while in this first phase.

2 **Starchy** vegetables ½ cup as serving size (Organic, fresh, non GMO and local if possible) Sweet potatoes, yams, beets, winter Winter, acorn or butternut squash, Jimica Parsnips, Taro (no white potatoes)

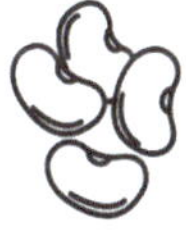

3 **Beans and legumes** - ½ cup as serving size (Organic, fresh, non GMO and local if possible) Azuki, Black, Black eyed peas, Cannelini, Fava, Garbanzo (Hummus), Great Northern, Kidney, Lima, Lentil, Mung, Navy, Pink, Pinto

4 **Animal based Proteins – no limitation** (Organic, grass fees, wild caught, local if possible) Chicken, Turkey, Lamb, Beef, Veal, Wild game, Buffalo, Rabbit, Venison, Fish, Tuna, Sardines, Tuna, Eggs

- Meat - Preferably, grass fad and organic
- Fish - Wild caught, free dyes (not farmed)
- Eggs – cage-free and free rage or on Pasture
- Pork – only if it is grass fed and organic

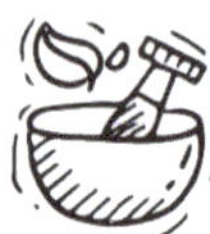

5 Herbs and Spices – no limitation (Organic, fresh, non GMO and local if possible) Anise, Alfalfa Sprouts, Basil, Bay, Cardamom, Chervil, Chili, Chives, Cinnamon, Cloves, Coriander leaf, Coriander seed, Cumin, Curry powder, Dill weed, Garlic, Ginger, Ginseng, Lavender, Lemon Grass, Mace,Marjoram, Nutmeg, Onion, Oregano, Paprika, Parsley, Pepper black, Peppermint, Rosemary, Saffron, Sage, Savory, Tarragon, Thyme, Turmeric

- Use liberally when cooking to flavor your food

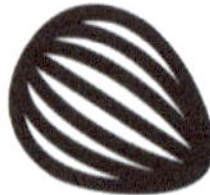

6 Nuts and Seeds – Raw only, no limitation (Organic, fresh, non GMO and local if possible) Walnuts, hazelnuts, filberts pecans, almonds, macadamia nuts, Brazil nut, cashews, flax seeds, chia seeds pumpkin seeds, sunflower seeds, poppy seeds sesame seeds – whole or as nut butters

You can also choose almond butter, cashews butter, Sesame past (thaini)

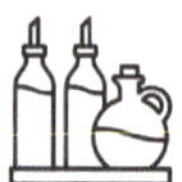

7 Fats and Oils - 6-8 teaspoons a day (Organic, fresh, non GMO and local if possible)

- Oils – olive oil, flax oil, grape seeds oils, avocado oil, almond oil, walnut oil, coconut oil, sesame oil, safflower, pumpkin oil

- Fats – butter, ghee, lard - unless specify differently

- Avocado – no limitation - unless specify differently

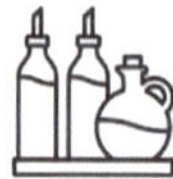

8 Lemon and lime juices - no limitation (Organic, fresh, non GMO and local if possible)

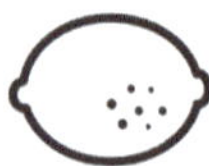

9 Liquid – Water, herbal tea (organic if possible. Warm or cold with NO SUGAR), You should drink eight glasses of water a day, 8-10 oz each

- Coffee - limit your intake to one or two cups a day (8oz max). Drink it plain NO cream or sugar or sweeteners.

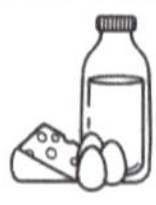

10 Dairy - Avoid at this stage. Dairy has lactose a form of sugar

BOTANICAL SUPPLEMENTS REQUIRED

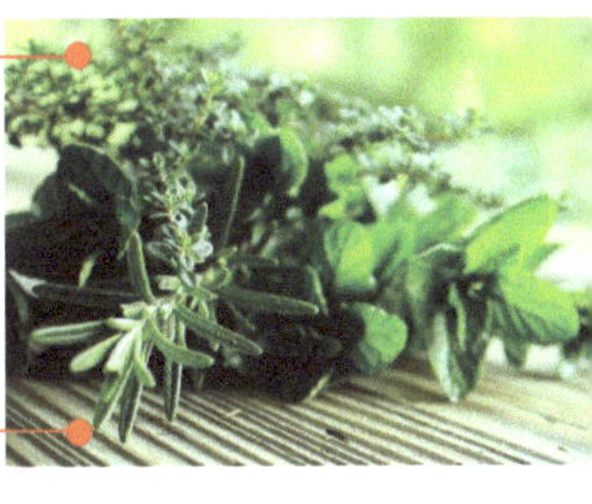

The botanical supplements are designed to provide your body with a complex of powerful phytonutrient like Biocidin, Oregano Oil, Olive Leaf Extract, Uva Ursi, Caprylic Acid, Allimax, glutamine, N-Acetyl Glucosamine, Marshmallow, Berberine, Slippery Elm and more for restoring and maintaining a healthy and balanced gastrointestinal microflora.

You want to includes ingredients that support the integrity of the gut, promote microbial balance, antioxidant protection, nourishing and soothing the intestinal cells, repair and maintain the mucosal barrier, as well as support normal inflammatory response.

Nutrient cofactors like minerals, trace minerals and vitamins are necessary to support the body's own production of HCL (Hydrochloric Acid - an acidifying compound normally produced by the stomach during digestion of foods. Promotes optimal gastric acidity to support protein digestion and absorption of minerals and other nutrients) which strengthen the protection of the stomach mucosal lining.

Biotin, is another crucial nutrient that inhibit yeast from changing into the aggressive fungal form.

Fatty acids like undecylenic and caprylic acid are powerful potent ingredients to disrupt the metabolism of candida and create a hostile environment for colonization.

Zinc Undecylenate is an additional nutrient you want to consider. Zinc Undecylenate inhibit the morphogenesis of Candida albicans; the compound also appears to interfere with fatty acid biosynthesis, inhibiting germ tube (hyphae) formation and disrupting the pH in yeast cells.

Binding agents like activated Charcoal, Flax seeds, Apple Pectin, Fiber binds to the "die-off" toxins. Increase bowel ovement

Probiotics must be included in your candida protocol. However, probiotic alone will NOT reduce the colonization of these opportunistic pathogens. The quality and the diversity of species used in the formulawill make a big different on how you will be able to control and reduce, our levels of candida infection.

Studies demonstrated that Lactobacillus GG, L. acidophilus, and Saccharomyces boulardi are the most effective with L. GG demonstrating the ability to induce antibody formation

against Candida. Not to say, healing various pathological conditions in the gastro-intestinal tract, when Candida is present.

The effectiveness of probiotics has been shown to decrease the presentation of Candida overgrowth in children, adults and the elderly population. According to this data, probiotics promote and stimulate the host immune response against intestinal Candida overgrowth and accelerate healing in the intestinal mucosa. In most of the studies, probiotics were used alongside antifungals not instead of.

Do not supplement yourself without a practitioner's supervision that has clinical experience and evaluates you, your current health and your present starting point. Nutrition nor Supplements alone will NOT take care of the Candida infection.

Please Note:

The above listed supplements are NOT the complete botanical supplements needed to decrease presentation of Candida overgrowth. Be sure to consult your health practitioner prior to any intervention.

"DIE-OFF" SYMPTOMS

Not all individuals will face a "die-off" symptoms, though you want to know that the following symptoms might happen. This is part of a healthy and positive process. It happens due to a release of toxins products into the bloodstream. When "killing" candida,

79 different toxics substance like acetaldehyde and ethanol will be released into the blood. Often, we need further adjustments to the initial protocol proposed.

Remember, the "die off" will slow down and even diminish over time.

The length and the severity of the symptoms depending on your:

- Candida Infection
- Liver health to detoxify
- Strong Immune system

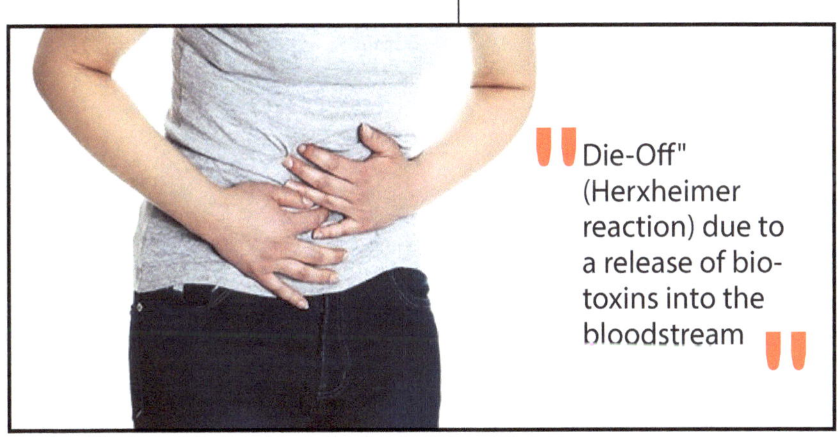

"DIE-OFF" SYMPTOMS POSSIBLE:

- Headache
- Brain Fog
- Nausea
- Fatigue
- Irritability
- Moodiness
- Digestive bloating and gas
- Fever
- Diarrhea, loose stools or constipation
- Rashes or itching
- Hyperactivity, restless
- Sleep disturbance

Dealing with Candida "Die-Off"

The above listed symptoms may last for few hours or few weeks. If you cannot tolerant the symptoms here are few steps you can take:

1. Consult your practitioner

2. Slow down or even cut back the antifungal supplements. The supplements taken are to break down the Biofilm of the candida (The walls of the Candida Yeast Cells). When this happens, more toxins are released into the blood. When get better, you can go back to the fully subscribed dosage.

It is better NOT to cut back ONLY if it is Impossible to tolerant the "Die-Off"

3. Increase water, herbal teas intakes

4. Increase vegetables intake (mainly warm cooked)

5. Increase protein and fats intake

6. Increase herbs like: cilantro, basil, parsley, dill.

7. If needed, rest, slow down (remember, it is only for few hours or days)

8. Your practitioner might add additional liver and immune support supplement

Always consult with your practitioner if symptoms are hard to tolerance.

FOOD LOG

	MON	TUES	WED	THU	FRO	SAT	SUN
BREACKFAST							
SNACK							
LUNCH							
SNACK							
DINNER							
SNACK							
LIQUID							
SLEEP							
BM							
NOTE							

This form is to keep track on: food portion, food quality, liquid intake, quality of sleep, volume of bowel movement (BM) and body's reacti on to new food

2

FOOD INTRODUCTION AND EVALUATION

30 - 60 days
Starting Date:

At this stage we want to re-introduce many of the foods that we eliminated in phase one. As well as, increase back food's volume of the 3 sub-groups that we limited in phase one; fruits, starchy vegetables and grains since they turn to be sugars which feed the candida.

It is highly recommended to do the IgG food allergy test to reduce any potential risk for immune reaction to foods that may have caused your parasitic infection. Regardless if you have

Food allergy test or not, you want to follow the next steps:

1 Instructions for Reintroducing Foods

Reintroducing the foods you eliminate from your diet is our next phase in our program achieving your health goals. Add one portion of one new food a day. In order to assess any reactions to those "new" foods you eliminated, the following is the suggested reintroducing procedure:

- Ingest the food you are reintroducing 2 to 3 times in the same day.

- Continue to eat the other foods on your diet.

- Do not introduce any other new foods over the next 3 days

- Monitor any reaction you may experience over the next 3 days

Possible Reactions:

Digestion/Bowel Function; Headache; Brain Fogginess, Nasal or Chest Congestion; Skin; Energy level; Joint /Muscle pain, Fatigue, Irritability, Moodiness, Fever, Sleep interruption, Blood Sugar elevating of >20 points (if monitoring)

- Wait 3 days
- On the third day you can reintroduce same food again
- Monitor your reaction, again

If your body shows no reactions:

If your body shows any reactions to any new food stop immediately and report back.

If you don't notice any reaction, continue to the second group of food and observe your body's response.

Please follow the following order when introducing back foods that were eliminated to reduce your infection:

Fruits, will be the first group of foods to be introduced back.

Starchy Vegetables will be the second group

Grains will be the last group of food you want to introduce back.

The order and or the rhythm might change based on your body's respond to the new group foods.

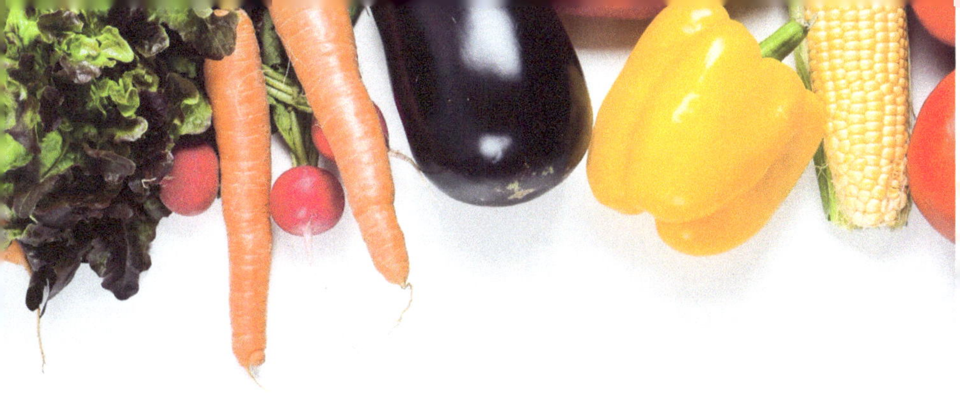

2   Food introduction oder:

1. Fruits – increase volume from ¼ cup to ½ cup 2-3 times in the challenged day.

2. Introduce only one type of fruit and watch for your body's response.

3. Starch Vegetables - increase volume from ½ cup to 1 cup 2-3 times in the chal lenged day. Introduce only one type of starchy vegetable and watch for your body's response.

4. Grains - increase volume from ½ cup to ¾ cup 2-3 times in the challenged day.

5. Introduce only one type of grain and watch for your body's response. Better to start with gluten free grains first like: Quinoa, Teff, Farro, Millet, Buckwheat, Sorghum, Amaranth rather than introducing wheat grain.

6. One food at the time. NO combination, No 2 different foods from 2 or more groups of foods.

IT IS A SLOW AND GRADUATE PROCESS – BE PATIENCE

Record the foods you eat while introducing back the foods as well as, your body's symptoms so you and your practitioner could link the symptoms with the status of your parasitic infection.

MAINTENANCE – ENJOY LIFE WITH THE NUTRITIONAL AND COOKING SKILLS YOU GAINED

You have learned so much about your body and how food and nutrition can affect your health. Yes, now is the time that you can loosen up a bit and avoid only those foods that either alert your symptoms by activating your immune system and or that you find yourself sensitive or allergic to them.

Try to balance, do not sabotage your body as well as your intestine bacterial flora by going back to old habits of the SAD (Standard American Diet) diet.An excess of any food (healthy or not) that is high in carbohydrates or sugar content will take you back to the starting point.

Moderation and Diversion of food are the key for maintaining and supporting normal inflammatory response, repairing and maintaining healthy mucosal barrier.

HEALTHY MEALS IDEAS TO CONTROL CANDIDA YEAST OVERGROWTH

One of the challenges most individuals will face during the first phase is following the nutritional changes to control their Candida Yeast Overgrowth.

We've put together some Candida Nutritional Meals Ideas to ease the process for you the best we could offer.

Just remember, this meal plan protocol is low in sugars and carbohydrates, which can lead to sugar and carbohydrates cravings at first. However, the craving will be balanced if you will eat enough proteins, fats and vegetables. When hungry you may increase your protein portion size.

This is not a calorie-restricted protocol. You have to nourish your body by eating properly. Foods that will support you to control Candida Yeast Overgrowth on one hand while keeping energy production, liver detoxification and inflammation reduction.

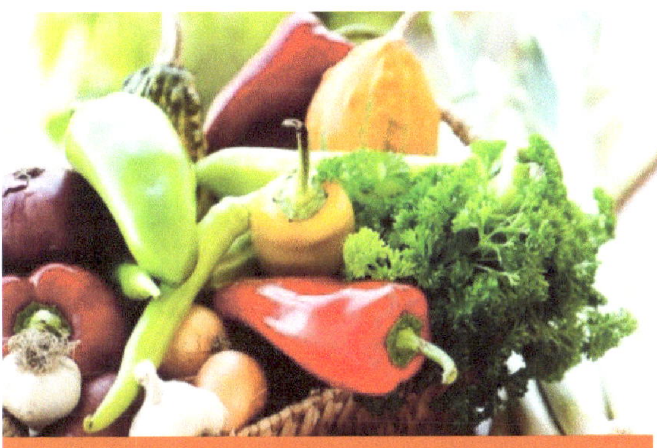

Please note that the suggested meals are general meal ideas. If you are SENSETIVE or Allergic to any proposed food (ingredient) you may want to AVOID or SUBSTITUTE it with another option to support your health.

BREAKFAST – LUNCH - DINNER

MEALS IDEAS

Eggs

- Hard (soft)-boiled

- Poached or

- Scrambled eggs with Vegetables like: spinach, onions, parsley, basil, kale, leeks, peppers (NO MUSHROOMS)

- Scrambled eggs with Spices like: cumin seeds, coriander, thymine, oregano, black pepper, anise seeds, Allspice, bay leaf, caraway, rosemary, sage, cloves, mustard, red pepper, turmeric ginger.

Soups

Soup is a super great comfort food, warming and easy to make, a perfect addition to support you in the process of controling your Candida Overgrowth. Most soups will provide you with many antioxidants, vitamins, mineral and fibers.

The key ingredients to make any soup recipe a winner soup, nourishing your body while healing your intestines lining is the broth (chicken or vegetable broth). If you do not make your own broth, please buy organic, non GMO, gluten free and no MSG product.

Oregano, cilantro, parsley, thyme, basil, dill are all great source of antibacterial components. As well as spices like: coriander, cloves, masala, turmeric, cumin, curry, ginger and garlic (if possible).

Use fresh organic herbs and spices to upgrade your soup flavors and healing properties.

Soups Ideas:

- Chicken Vegetables soup
- Vegetable Cabbage-Parsley Soup
- Cauliflower-Ginger Soup
- Broccoli-Coconut Milk Soup
- Jerusalem Artichoke Soup
- Minestrone Soup (no tomatoes)
- Fennel-Dill Soup
- Asparagus-Onion-Leek Soup
- Carrots-Cilantro Soup

You can increase to any recipe additional portions of proteins like chicken, turkey, beef, eggs and even fish so you can add more calories. Beans, lentils, and starchy vegetables will break down to sugars due to the carbohydrate content. You want to limit the quantity of
these food to no more than ½ cup (4oz) as a serving size.

LUNCH AND DINNER RECIPES

Creating your new meals will support you in controlling Candida Overgrowth. Remember, you need to eat plenty of proteins (animal and/or plant base), healthy fats and vegetables to feel satisfy. If not satisfied, most likely you will go back to grains, carbohydrates, sweets and fruits.

Try to stay away from processed food and alcohol as much as you can (at least in phase 1 and 2)

Here are some tasty lunch and dinner ideas that can support you in controlling your candida.

Grilled Lamb

(or breast chicken or beef or turkey) with baked cauliflower
(or any other vegetable)

Mix greens Salads

(lettuce, kale, spinach, arugula, chard, collard, freisse, radicchio greens) with:

○ Grilled breast chicken or beef or lamb or turkey

○ Grilled Salmon or cod or tuna or sardines or anchovies or Herring or Cooked beans

○ Avocado, artichoke, Jerusalem artichoke

○ Roasted beets, asparagus, cauliflower, broccoli, Brussel sprouts, Bok Choy, string green string beans

○ Eggs

○ Nuts and seeds

○ Feta cheese, blue cheese

Yogurt

cow's milk (Greek yogurt), goat milk or kefir with:

○ Cucumber, green onion, avocado and one of the following fresh herbs like: basil, dill, parsley, mint Basil, cloves, chives – drizzle with olive oil (or any other oil), lemon and salt

Vegetables-Proteins Wraps

use chard, kale or iceberg lettuces as you wrap base. Top with grilled chicken, lamp strips, tuna, salmon, avocado, roasted vegetables (onions, peppers, zucchini), add some arugula, basil or oregano leafs. Roll and eat.

Again, this are only meal ideas. You surely can create your own following the guides provided.

REFERENCES

1. Arch Intern Med. 1989 Apr;149(4):962-4. Candidal sinusitis and diabetic

2. ketoacidosis. A brief report. Dooley DP1, McAllister CK

3. Am J Med Sci. 1990 Jun;299(6):379-85. Effect of prolonged modified fasting in obese persons on in vitro markers of immunity: lymphocyte function and serum effects on normal neutrophils. McMurray RW1, Bradsher RW, Steele RW, Pilkington NS.

4. A Watson in 1976, J. Bacteriol; M Lopez and C Silva in 1984, Z. Allg. Mikrobiol 24; V.

5. Uden and H. Buckley in 1970, The Yeasts; Lemos-Carolino and Madeira-Lopes in

6. 1984, Sabouraudia 22.

7. 4. Andoni Ramirez-Garcia, Aitor Rementeria, Jose Manuel Aguirre-Urizar, Maria Dolores Moragues, Aitziber Antoran, Aize Pellon, Ana Abad-Diaz-de-Cerio, and Fernando Luis Hernando, Candida albicans and cancer: Can this yeast induce cancer development or progression? Critical Reviewing in Microbiology, Informs Health Care, January,

8. 2014

9. 5. Antimicrob Agents Chemother. Jul 2004; 48(7): 2350–2354.

10. Crook, WG. The Yeast Connection Handbook. Jackson, Tennessee: Professional

11. Books, Inc.; 2002.

12. Crook, WG, Cass H. The Yeast Connection and Women's Health. Jackson, Tennessee:

13. Professional Books, Inc.; 2003.

14. Leyla Muedin is a clinical nutritionist and lecturer at the Hoffman Center and is available for speaking engagements for private and public sector wellness programs

15. "Candidiasis." March 8, 2001. CDC. <http://cdc.gov/ncidod/bdmd/disease info/can didacies-t.htm>

16. Clinkscales, Cynthia. Healthy at Last: Solutions to chronic ill health, allergies and environmental illness. Arkansas: CECOM, 1990.

17. Galland, MD., Leo. "The Effect of Intestinal Microbes on Systemic Immunity." 1998.

18. Microbes.

19. Importance of some factors on the dimorphism of Candida albicans. Vidotto V1, Picerno G, Caramello S, Paniate G. Mycopathologia 1988 Dec;104(3):129-35.

20. Introduction; Paragraph 2, first sentence: "Biotin is required by a variety of yeasts, fungi and bacteria, not only for growth but also for metabolite production".

21. Iralu, Appl. Microbial 22, 1971 and CE Webster, FC Odds J. Med. Vet. Mycol. 25, 1987.

22. Kaufmann, Doug A. The Fungus

Link: An introduction to fungal disease including the initial phase diet. Ed. Beverly Thornhill Hunt, Ph.D. Texas: Media Trition, 2000.

23. Knox, BA DC, Dr. Jerry Glenn. Candida. Washington: Lifeknox, 2002

24. "Medical Encyclopedia" May 2, 2005. Medline Plus. <http://www. nlm.nih.gov/med lineplus/ency/ article/000964.htm>

25. Meyer SA, Ahearn DG, Yarrow DG, published in Elsevier Science Publ. in 1984.

26. Tissue invasiveness and non-acidic pH in human candidiasis correlate with "in vivo" expression by Candida albicans of the carbohydrate epitope recognized by new monoclonal antibody 1H4. Tissue invasiveness and non-acidic pH in human candidi asis correlate with "in vivo" expression by Candida albicans of the carbohydrate epitope recognized by new monoclonal antibody 1H4. – Journal of Clinical Patholo gy. 2004 Jun; 57(6): 598–603. doi: http://www. ncbi.nlm.nih.gov/pmc/articles/P MC1770313/

27. "The Fourth NIAID Workshop in Medical Mycology: Host Responses to Fungi." NIAID

28. January 5, 2001. <http://www.niaid. nih.gov/dmid/meetings/mycology97/ immuno.htm>

29. "THE INTERACTION OF MICROORGANISMS WITH THE COMPLEMENT SYSTEM: FUNGI." October 21, 2004. Microbiology @ Leicester.

30. <http://www-micro.msb.le.ac.uk/ MBChB/Merralls/Fungi.html>

31. Sauer, Gordon C. The Manual of Skin Diseases, 6th Ed. Philadelphia: J.B. Lippincott

32. Co., 1991.

33. "What is Candida?" 2004. Ninazu Health Products Inc.

34. <http://www.ninazu.com/whatis. html>

35. "Yeast Infections." McGraw-Hill Encyclopedia of Science and Technology. 9th Ed.

36. Vol.19. New York: McGraw-Hill Co. Inc., 2002.

37. http://www.ncbi.nlm.nih.gov/pmc/ articles/PMC3084579/

ABOUT THE AUTHOR

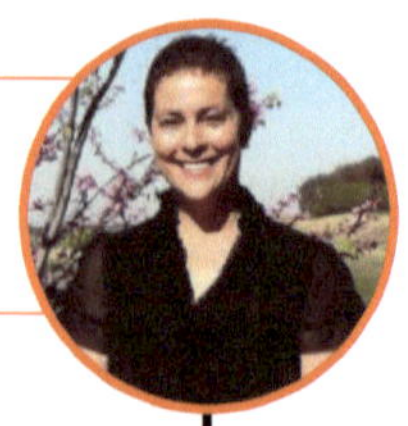

Chen Ben Asher, a clinician, public speaker, educator and author of Amazon Best Seller – "What If Gluten Free Is Not Enough". She uses Functional Nutrition to help you find answers to the root causes of your illness and address the biochemical imbalances that may trigger your health and weight. She uses cutting edge lab testing and design the nutritional program to your specific needs as an individual. Food, supplements, lifestyle changes will have integrated to bring balance.

If you are looking for personalized nutritional support, we highly recommended contacting Mor's Nutrition & More Wellness Center in Cupertino, California today.

Food Intelligence

Chen provides nutritional care for those wanting to improve their quality of life through a gentle and effective diet. Chen brings more than 15 years of experience serving our community. Her effective, holistic nutritional approach will support you on your life's journey to achieve your body's optimal wellness by losing weight while gaining health.

 408.966.4972

 contact@mor-nutrition4life.com

 http://www.mor-nutrition4life.com

CANDIDA - FUNCTIONAL NUTRITION